CLARA MIA

Kama Sutra Book Of Sex Positions

Guide On How Discover New, Historical And Erotic Sex Positions To Spice Up Your Relationship And Sexual Life As a Beginner

Copyright © 2022 by Clara Mia

First edition

This book was professionally typeset on Reedsy
Find out more at reedsy.com

Contents

1. INTRODUCTION 1
2. SEVERAL BENEFITS OF INCREASING SEX IN A RELATIONSHIP..3
The Importance of Sex in Relationships..............................3
Benefits of Sexual Activity in Marriage................................3
Benefits of Sexual Activity for Mental Health 3
Physical Benefits of Having More Sex.................................3
Ideal Sexual Intervals 3
3. KAMA SUTRA SEX POSITIONS THAT BEGINNERS CAN DO 10
4. FOREPLAY SUGGESTIONS FROM KAMA SUTRA TO SPICE UP YOUR SEXUAL LIFE...18
5. HOW TO BUILD INTIMACY IN RELATIONSHIPS 21
6. COMMON SEXUAL FANTASIES 34
7. HOW TO GIVE YOUR PARTNER A HOT SENSUAL MASSAGE 41
Tips for swiftly and practically performing a pleasant massage 41
8. FUN FOREPLAY SEX POSITIONS..49
9. HOW TO TALK DIRTY WITH YOUR PARTNER DURING SEX..55
10. CONCLUSION 60
   1.
   2.
      1.
      2.

3.
4.
5.
3.
4.
5.
6.
7.
1.
8.
9.

One

INTRODUCTION

The Kama Sutra may have come on your radar. That's because the Indian philosopher Vatsyayanas Kama sutra, which serves as a manual for essentially all sex positions, has attracted a lot of attention. The Kama Sutra has been widely translated and used in the West, particularly in the United States. Considering sexuality and the colonial foundations of modern social theories, incorrect translation.

Statecraft, urban life, scents, and horticulture were all included in the original collection of writings that is now known as the Kama sutra. Richard Button, an orientalist and proponent of colonialism, translated the Kama Sutra into English for the first time in the late nineteenth century, which led to the text's distortion. Burton tried to create a fantasy for his English-speaking audience by depicting easterners as hypersexual, immutable, and without history. Unfortunately, both historical and modern language still perpetuates these restrictive, prejudiced notions about Indian sexuality. Sex positions are discussed in the Kama Sutra, albeit only briefly. It's all about the art of enjoying life to the fullest, which includes finding love, having sex, and spice up your sexual life.

However, there are many sex positions in the sexuality area that encourage emotional connection between partners through verbal, nonverbal, and physical cues. Even ancient literature advises men to prioritize a woman's pleasure by making sure she is aroused before considering having an orgasm of their own. The Kama Sutra's sexuality chapter was written to instruct a gentleman on how to make sure that the woman was perfectly satisfied. They believed that sex would last longer in a relationship if a woman was completely satisfied, and that if a man could successfully win a woman's respect.

The target audience for this book includes established couples, individuals wishing to date, and people looking to spice up their relationships and sexual life. It is for those who wish to work on more than simply the sexual component of their relationship.

Two

SEVERAL BENEFITS OF INCREASING SEX IN A RELATIONSHIP

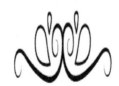

There are several benefits to increasing sex in a supportive relationship. Higher rates of sexual activity are linked to beneficial changes including lower blood pressure, less stress, more intimacy, and even a lower divorce rate. Even though there are no universally accepted rules for the ideal sex frequency, I have shared insight from the most recent studies.

Its chapter also discusses the data on the frequency of sexual activity between partners, the justifications for this significance, some potential benefits, and the significance of sex in relationships. Even conceivable challenges you can face as a sexual partner are covered, along with suggestions for how to encourage sex in your relationship.

The Importance of Sex in Relationships

Can a relationship endure without sexual activity? Yes. Sex is not always necessary. It might, however, be an important element of a fulfilling, lasting relationship.

Sex may or may not matter to a particular person. Some people might think it's imperative to be in a sexual relationship. Some individuals might think that other types of intimacy and connection are more important.

The following factors may lead you to believe that having sex is essential in a relationship:

- having a stronger sense of partnership
- demonstrating love for your spouse
- enjoying sex and having the desire to have children while feeling seductive and powerful
- lowering of tension

Having frequent intercourse may have an impact on a person's general wellbeing. It is well known that having sex makes people more affectionate. As a couple's level of affection rises, the likelihood of them having more frequent sex rises.

Benefits of Sexual Activity in Marriage

Beyond the benefits it offers for you and your partner individually, regular sex promotes a good relationship in a number of ways. For instance, the oxytocin produced during intercourse enhances bonding and emotional connection.

In a monogamous relationship, sex deepens your emotional connection and level of commitment. When a couple expresses their love sexually, they are more likely to stay together. Therefore, sex is positively associated with a lower divorce rate.

Benefits of Sexual Activity for Mental Health

Numerous psychological and emotional benefits result from romantic love (sex is strongly linked to a better quality of life). These benefits comprise, among others:

Sexual activity can improve self-worth and reduce insecurity, which leads to more positive assessments of oneself.

Higher satisfaction rates are correlated with greater amounts of consenting sex and higher caliber sex.

More kinship Endorphins, which are released during sexual activity, reduce irritability and depression symptoms. The hormone oxytocin (commonly referred to as the "hug drug") increases with nipple stimulation and other sexual activity. Oxytocin helps to develop a calm and contented state of mind.

Taking a stress break Long-term stress may make people have less sex as often. However, having sex can help you cope with stress.

During sexual activity, the stress response hormones cortisol and adrenaline (epinephrine) are lowered, and the effects last far into the next day.

Orgasms cause the production of the sleep-inducing hormone prolactin, which leads to better-quality sleep.

Physical Benefits of Having More Sex

Although it should be clear how having sex improves emotional wellness, there are also a number of physical benefits. Here are a handful of them:

- **Better physical fitness:** Sex is a physical activity. Sexual activity is comparable to light exercise, such brisk walking or climbing two flights of steps. During intercourse, the muscles in the abdomen and pelvis may tone up and tighten. Women who exercise regularly have greater bladder control.
- **Better cognitive function** and the generation of new brain cells have been linked to higher internet connectivity and sexual engagement in preliminary rat studies. Similar benefits have since been discovered in human studies. In a study with over 6,000 participants, regular sex was linked to improved memory in persons over 50.
- The health of the immune system is positively impacted by increased sexual activity.

Sex on a regular basis may even lower your chance of catching the flu or a cold.

- **Decreased levels of pain:** Sex-related endorphins have effects beyond simply promoting relaxation and well-being. Additionally, it appears that sex endorphins ease headache and back pain.
- **Weight loss:** Sex normally burns 200 calories in a 30-minute session. The pleasant brain chemicals that are generated during sex can help with weight loss by lowering food cravings.
- **Health benefits:** Penile-vaginal sexual activity, but not masturbation, has been linked to lower systolic blood pressure. 11 Elevated blood pressure increases the risk of both heart disease and stroke. Sexual activity decreases blood pressure and improves the circulation of nutrients and oxygen throughout the body by expanding blood vessels.
- **Additional physical benefits**, such as a rise in desire and enhanced vaginal lubrication brought on by increased sexual activity. Less painful cramps and shorter menstrual cycles are associated with regular sexual activity. Additionally, the body's release of the hormone DHEA during an orgasm may be linked to improved digestion, healthier teeth, a better sense of smell, and glowing skin.

Ideal Sexual Intervals

A study found that when considering how frequently a couple should have sex, sexual frequency is, to a limited extent, connected to general well-being.

From no sex until once a week, relationship satisfaction grew gradually, but after that, it stopped rising (and even started to decline slightly). The weekly average of one sexual encounter is currently pretty consistent. However, due of how busy our lives are, we might not be able to have more sex. In comparison to the previous year, adults had sexual activity nine fewer times each year.

Although the frequency of sexual activity tends to decrease with age, it is still important in older people. In general, older married couples had more sexual encounters than their single age-group counterparts.

The typical sexual frequency

An adult typically has 54 periods every year (about once per week)

20-something adults: About 80 times per year.

Adults over 60: 20 times per year

Increased Chances of Sexual Activity

It was long believed that having sex increased a man's risk of prostate cancer. However, a study discovered that men who ejaculated more regularly (21 or more times per month) had a lower risk of contracting the condition than those who did not (seven or less per month). Because prostate cancer is the second leading cause of cancer-related deaths in men, it is crucial to be aware of this consequence.

Some people's chance of having a heart attack increases as a result of having sex. Even with this danger, regular sex might be advantageous. Heart attacks are less likely when people have regular sex. Both sex and other physical activity are protective. However, brief bouts of exercise more frequently strain the heart. Speak with your doctor about your sexual behavior to determine your risks.

Challenges of Regular Sex

There is no denying the significance of sex in a relationship, but there are a lot of factors that might make being a sexual couple more challenging. Age, hormones, children, stress, sicknesses, and relationship problems are just a few of the variables that might influence a couple's frequency of sex.

How frequently people have sex is significantly influenced by the decline in sex hormone levels that happens as people age.

Sometimes, problems with one's physical or mental health make maintaining an active sex life difficult or impossible. Humans are driven by the intimacy of sex. Absence of sex can cause partners in a relationship to grow distant and even search elsewhere. By meeting with a trained couples therapist, you may bridge this gap and stop issues from impacting your marriage.

Three

KAMA SUTRA SEX POSITIONS THAT BEGINNERS CAN DO

•69 (Position)

The Kama Sutra places a high value on giving pleasure, and what better way to accomplish it than with a little oral adoration? Pleasure and the anticipation of pleasure are topics that are covered throughout the Kama Sutra. You may get a good start on foreplay by making your spouse and yourself both feel good. Place cushions under your butt so that your spouse can reach you from a variety of angles. By changing the angles, you can alter your feelings and increase your level of pleasure.

Try it: Do this while lying flat on your back. Then, while keeping their backs to your upper body, have your partner climb to the top. Your partner's mouth should be lined up with your genitalia, and their genitalia should be lined up with theirs. (You can alter positions to try out other points of view.)

•Face off (position)

You have complete control over every aspect of this circumstance because you are in charge, including the tempo, angle, and depth. The only portion of your body that can move when on top, according to the Kama Sutra, is your hips. If you move more than just your hips, your back could suffer. To keep the focus on the pleasure, try to isolate your actions.

Try It: While your partner is perched on a chair or the edge of a bed, sit on their lap and face them.

•Champagne room (position)

The benefit of being seated is that you are once again in control. The Kama Sutra placed a lot of emphasis on allowing women to wear jewelry that might act as a guide for them when engaging in sex. For seated positions, you wore a seven- or nine-string pearl necklace. "You want the pearls to move very lightly from side to side…the body movement will just flow," you were instructed. Try reclining and slightly raising your hips so that your partner's knees are bearing the weight of your body.

Try It: Sit on top of your partner while facing away. Your partner should take a seat.

•Pretzel Dip (position)

Look each other in the eyes and enjoy the pleasures of doggy style in this cute, food-inspired pose. Make it a sensual experience by petting your partner's buttocks, reaching around to touch their nipples and breasts, and clitoral stimulation to heighten the enjoyment in this position. By playing with different angles until you discover the one that works best for you, you may amp things up even further.

Try it: Do as advised and lie on your right side. Your partner straddles your right leg while kneeling and wrapping their left leg around their left side.

•Spork (Position)

Make lots of eye contact and utilize a seductive Kama Sutra method to perfume various regions of your body while you bump and grind in the spork pose. Every portion of the body had to be "fragranced with a distinct perfume," according to the Kama Sutra. Your partner is virtually drawn to your body as you transform into a feast of flavors, textures, and scents.

Try It: Lay on your back and elevate your right leg to provide a 90-degree angle for your partner to squeeze between your knees as you. To alter the depth of penetration, you can either bend your left leg or extend it straight out over the bed. For a rear-entry alternative, lie on your stomach, bend one leg, and have your partner crawl between your thighs.

• **Cowgirls Helper (position)**

Here, the face-to-face component is fantastic. Try discussing and exchanging dreams while having sex, yes "for the most intimate experience possible. "To increase closeness, I'll advise you to kiss, lock eyes, and stroke your partner's nipples.

Try It: This is a small variation on the cowgirl sex position. As you kneel on top of your lover, you push off their chest and slide up and down their thighs. As they rise to meet each thrust, your partner assists by bearing some of your weight and holding onto your hips or thighs.

• **Doggy Style**

You're not exactly face to face when you do it doggy style, but there's a cool solution: Use a mirror. Looking in the mirror can aid with the presence of the sexual experience, as well as eroticism and pleasure. There is also a very strong trust emotion that arises from doing this because the person in the "doggy" position is in a passive, defenseless position. You and your significant other "come in line with the Kama Sutra as they are allowing for diverse sorts of pleasure-giving and receiving to and for each other as they are doing in either scenario,"

Get on all fours and give it a try. After that, have your partner squat behind you with their upper body either straight up or partially draped over yours.

- **G-whiz (position)**

If you and your partner aren't particularly flexible, this motion is a great alternative for you. If you and your partner are different heights, you can use a sex cushion or place some pillows underneath the other person.

Try It: While your partner is sat on their knees, lie back with your legs resting on their shoulders.

- **The Magic mountain (position)**

This scissor-like technique works well for girl-on-girl sex since lovers can physically enthrall one another with a toy or their hands.

Try It: Have your partner sit with their knees bent and lean back on their hands and forearms. Then, until you make contact, you do the same as them.

- **The Chairman (position)**

This is another situation where you can feel like bouncing is appropriate, but I usually suggest grinding. A great opening move for nipple play, deep penetration, and having your partner kiss your shoulders and neck is the chairman.

Want to take it to the next level? Asking your partner to touch you will manual arouse you when you are holding a sex object.

Try it: Sit on top of your partner as they are sitting on the edge of the bed.

- **The pinball wizard (position)**

A top-notch Kama Sutra maneuver for thorough penetration, this one. If you are unable to maintain the bridge position or your partner is unable to support your lower body with their arms, you might want to try another exercise (because over-exertion is not sexy).

Try it: Get into a pinball-like partial bridge position where your shoulders are bearing the majority of your weight. Your sweetheart kneels down and walks over to you.

- **The good EX (position)**

This close-quarters position is easier than it seems. This is a great opportunity for you to utilize a vibrating wand on yourself at the same time. And for added pleasure, anyone who is rocking back and forth while seated can also consider using a butt plug.

Try It: Your legs should be extended and facing each other while you sit on the bed. Your left partner should elevate his left leg over your right leg as you do. Allow him to enter both of you. You are both currently lying back, your legs forming an X. Instead of thrusting, there are leisurely, languid gyrations. Hello proximity!

- **Ballet dancer (position)**

If it becomes difficult for you and your partner to stay balanced while in this sex position, try not to lose patience. Swap directions instead. You can give that person a cunnilingus or blow job by getting down on your knees, or the opposite. The most crucial factor is that you made an effort.

Try It: Face your spouse while standing on one foot and crossing your other leg over their waist as they support you.

•The Reverse cowgirl

Due to the inherent curve of most strap-ons or penises, this one is a little difficult, but it is still possible. (It is understandable why ladies are against this sex position.) It's fun once you get your rhythm, though.

Tip: I typically advise putting a pillow under each knee to increase your range of motion when you're on top.

Try it: Straddle your partner while they are on their back and facing their feet.

•Stand and deliver (position)

If you're feeling very bold, try the Stand and Deliver. The Kama Sutra approves of this technique, which already works well for shallow penetration. If you want deeper penetration, you can instead bring it to your knees. This adjustment is an excellent way to take into consideration differences in height. If you're the one on the receiving end and worried about collapsing as things get heated, I always suggest leaning on a table or a chair for support.

Try It: Bend down at the waist while you're still standing and let them enter from behind.

•Missionary (position)

One of the most underrated professions is missionary. Even if it's straightforward, doing so will nonetheless make you feel closer to your partner—after all, the Kama Sutra mentions this very thing. Due to the frequent close eye contact, the "feels," and the "so many various permutations," it is extremely intimate.

Try placing cushions beneath your pelvis to force your lover on top to thrust upward diagonally, grating into your clitoris.

Try It: Lie on your back with your partner lying face down on top of you.

Four

FOREPLAY SUGGESTIONS FROM KAMA SUTRA TO SPICE UP YOUR SEXUAL LIFE

Foreplay suggestions from the Kama Sutra to spice up your sexual life

The kama sutra has a very distinctive quality. In terms of advice and tricks, it has a number of aces up its sleeve. Both men and women can use the detailed guidance on sex, pleasure, and desire found in the ancient Vedic scripture to improve their sex lives. It goes beyond simple sexual action and doesn't stop there. You want your foreplay to be as delightful and sensual as it can be. So here are some foreplay tips from Kama sutra to make your time in bed more enjoyable!

•**Keep your partner close.**

First of all, it entails physical contact in addition to merely a hug. The flame will begin to rekindle and spread pleasure between the two of you as you engage in intimate contact. The prolonged touching period organically awakens you both, and an embrace like this strengthens your love for your spouse.

•**Close-mouth kisses**

Don't plunge in first. Take your time and carefully examine your partner's lips. As it gets slower and more sensuous, it gets more erogenous. Beginning with a soft kiss, gradually increase the intensity. This is the perfect way to trick your lover into thinking you want sex.

•**Use your nails to their full potential.**

Raking your nails across your partner's body after the kissing is finished will produce a wonderfully raw, seductive, and steamy feeling. Women love to massage their lovers' bodies, and when it gets heated and intense, they cling on tight!

•Attempt it!

Biting is highly thrilling sexually when done gently. Because chewing on the sensual spots substantially intensifies the sexual desire, it can be very stimulating for both of you. It is also intimately tied to the mechanics of dominance in bed.

•Honoring your spouse

When you submit to your lover as a symbol of authority, the sex session becomes immensely sexy and sensual. Both men and women have the capacity to alternately play the submissive. You can achieve your dreams in a variety of ways by increasing power. The ability to project a small amount of aggression and authority is really enticing and seductive.

Five

HOW TO BUILD INTIMACY IN RELATIONSHIPS

Intimacy is the term used to describe proximity between individuals in intimate relationships.

It's what grows through time as you get to know someone, grow to care for them, and feel more comfortable being with them.

It can include both emotional and physical intimacy, or even a mix of the two.

Priorities first: Intimacy and sex are distinct concepts.

You probably associate sex and romance with the word "intimacy" when you hear it.

For instance, having sex with someone is sometimes referred to as "being intimate." But intimacy and sex are not the same thing. It is possible to feel closeness without engaging in sexual activity, and vice versa.

It shouldn't be limited to just romantic or sexual partners, either. Although the first things that come to mind may be sex and romance, proximity is crucial in other sorts of relationships as well!

What do you mean, for example, when you say a "intimate gathering" is a party with friends? You're suggesting that a small group of close friends rather than a big number of strangers attended the celebration. You can also be discussing how effectively you used your time together. Perhaps you and your buddies grew closer as a result of having similar hobbies and sharing personal information.

Your relationships with your family, friends, and other trustworthy people depend on intimacy.

In the end, it means different things to different people.

While your date might be ready to go for a walk with you after the movie, you might feel closer to one another after you see a movie together. This is because everyone's notion of intimacy is different. How personal you think a connection is may depend on your preferences for meeting new people, your communication style, or other factors.

There are several types of intimacy as well.

Find out what intimacy means to you by considering the many types of intimacy.

There are several types of intimacy, such as:

•**Emotional**

Because of your emotional connection, you can disclose private information to your loved ones that you might not necessarily communicate with strangers. Think of it as letting your guard down. When you start to trust someone, you feel safe enough to relax your boundaries.

Do you anticipate spending quality time with your partner after work to relax and just be yourself? Or how can you talk to your brother without worrying about being rejected? Emotional connectivity appears like this.

•**Intellectual**

Sharing mental maps and understanding how others think are two aspects of intellectual intimacy.

It expands when you talk and have in-depth discussions. Do you recall that lengthy philosophical discussion that helped you to see that your classmate was more than simply a peer—he or she was also a friend? Or the first time you talked to your significant other all night long and felt the chemistry "spark"?

During these periods, you were intellectually close to one another, which made you more intimate.

•**Experiential**

You can create intimacy through spending time together and getting to know someone better through similar interests and hobbies.

Nothing comes close to the connection you make with someone over a game of Monopoly or while watching "Game of Thrones."

•**Physical**

Physical intimacy is primarily characterized by touch and closeness between bodies.

In a romantic relationship, it could entail holding hands, cuddling, kissing, and sexual activity. A warm, tight hug is an example of physical intimacy with a buddy.

•**Spiritual**

Varying people's definitions of spirituality will result in different amounts of spiritual connection.

The belief that there is something more important than the physical world is referred to as spirituality in general. This belief could be in a higher power, in human souls, or in a loftier objective, for example.

Spiritual connections can be demonstrated by sharing a common value, such as kindness, having the same opinions about organized religion, or feeling destined to be in each other's life.

Important components of any meaningful connection

All intimacy comes down to a few key components, like:

•**Trust**

To reveal private information about yourself, such as your most embarrassing secrets or your biggest fears, you must be able to trust the other person.

You might also strengthen your relationship with someone by proving your dependability to them.

•**Acceptance**

You have established some intimacy when you feel that someone accepts you for who you truly are.

You could be worried that if someone hears your "guilty pleasure" music playlist at a first meeting, they'll find you odd.

As closeness grows, though, you are free to rock out to your favorite boy bands and feel secure in the knowledge that your spouse will remain loyal to you whatever how bizarre you get.

•**Honesty**

Honesty and intimacy support one another. Often, one does not exist without the other. You and your partner have become so intimate that you feel comfortable sharing your feelings with them.

Similar to that, every time you open up, you can get a little bit closer. You'll know your spouse is willing to listen the next time you want to communicate something personal.

•**Safety**

When you show someone your most genuine self, you could feel quite vulnerable. Because of this, whenever you encounter new people, you frequently raise your guard. You don't yet know whether they will support you in the way that you are.

In other words, intimacy is the ability to put yourself out there with the assurance that the other person cares about you enough to keep their end of the bargain.

•Compassion

It's lovely to feel cared for, isn't it?

You know your best buddy would be there for you if you experienced a devastating split. You know that your sister won't keep you in the dark for more than a week before calling.

Forgiveness and understanding can only result from compassion amongst individuals.

When one cares about the welfare of another, compassion for them comes naturally.

•Affection

Being worried about one another is one thing, but showing that concern can also lead to intimacy.

Physical expressions of affection might include a hug, kiss, or embrace between lovers or a parent and kid, although they are not required.

Unconsciously, a friend shows their affection when they volunteer their free time to assist you move because they care.

•Communication

Effective communication is commonly mentioned as the cornerstone of a happy relationship for a reason.

When you make an effort to hear what they have to say and communicate your actual feelings, you can grow closer and more understanding.

And as you get to know one another better, your relationship gets stronger.

Intimacy rarely just happens; it usually needs to be built.

When you wake up one morning, you won't announce that you are now intimate. Got the job done!

More like a skill that you work on mastering through time, intimacy.

The more experiences and feelings you share with one another, the more tools you have at your disposal to foster intimacy.

Furthermore, it isn't always easy.

You could feel some apprehension or even anxiety when you establish connection.

That makes sense because intimacy demands opening up to another person and putting your trust in them despite the chance that they might let you down.

If someone has ever violated your confidence, it could take some time before you want to take a chance with them again.

Once you have it, though, your health may be dramatically impacted.

Since there is a probability of getting injured, why risk intimacy?

Well, being near has some health benefits that you simply cannot get any other way.

Deep friendship makes you feel like someone "gets" you and reduces feelings of loneliness.

Physical touch, such as hugs, and emotional release, such as laughter, activate your feel-good hormones, which improves your mental health by reducing stress.

In actuality, being near reduces the risk of heart disease, boosts the immune system, and decreases blood pressure.

It's a requirement for living a happy, healthy life.

How to get over an intimacy fear

If you're wary of closeness, you're not alone. It is doable to overcome it.

Here are some tips for getting over a fear of intimacy:

•Outline the circumstances and a list of your symptoms.

Although you might be conscious of your fear of intimacy, you might also be afraid of intimacy without even realizing it.

You might avoid long-term partnerships or struggle with social anxiety for unidentified reasons.

Do you shun social events and keep to yourself? have a negative self image? struggling to stay awake during sex? Do you not want others to know you?

Once you can spot a pattern, finding your symptoms might give you a specific list of things to work on.

Many people find it helpful to work with a therapist or other mental health professional to help them manage life.

•Set boundaries and explain why you have them.

You won't need to feel bad about it once you understand why you initially had your guard raised.

A dread of proximity might be a reasonable response to trauma, such as sexual assault or child mistreatment, for example.

We may try to isolate ourselves from the outside world after abuse in an effort to protect ourselves from judgment and further misery.

You can deliberately set the boundaries you want to keep and start to walk away from the ones that are no longer essential once you've identified what makes you feel safe and what makes you scared.

•Share your feelings with someone.

It can be difficult to establish trust with someone who isn't aware of your difficulties.

If you're married, you might confess to your partner that you struggle with vulnerability and that you're working on it.

If you feel comfortable enough to do so, you can also talk about your concerns and where they came from.

To feel confident in your relationships with the people in your life, it's appropriate to let them know what you expect of them.

•Obtain experienced assistance

Everybody periodically needs assistance facing their worries. A therapist or other mental health professional can offer that.

A professional can also assist you:

Find the cause of your aversion to closeness, deal with unpleasant issues like trauma, and assess your mental health for the presence of conditions like depression or avoidant personality disorder.

How to increase closeness in any form of relationship

Relationships frequently feel stagnant over time as life gets in the way and you fall into a rhythm that is less exciting than when you first met.

These ideas will assist you in rekindling or igniting intimacy in any relationship.

•Be sure to thank them for their help.

Spend some time telling the other person what you admire about them. Give them something, do something kind for them, or just say "thank you" to show your appreciation.

•Seek to learn more about one another.

After getting to know someone well, it could seem as though the "mystery" has been solved.

However, people and their relationships change and grow through time. There is always more to learn. To keep learning new things, play games like "20 Questions," swap stories, and ask questions. To genuinely understand the other person's worries and intentions, you must listen.

•Plan time specifically for your connection.

If you're not paying attention, time could pass without you having any important interactions.

Give it top priority as a result! Plan a weekly date night, a monthly board game night, or a daily minute to check in with each other before bed. Do this away from the kids or other responsibilities.

•Turn off devices and focus on one another.

When you spend time together without any technology, you may be able to give each other uninterrupted attention.

•Make warm eye contact (even without sex)

To avoid being bored in a sexual relationship, try adding new accessories, outfits, and fantasies.

Making it a point to show physical appreciation without engaging in sexual activity is another way to deepen connection.

Making loving gestures and snuggling can help you remember that joining your bodies together is for more than just "getting off."

•Combining forces on a project

Learn to bake, repair a piece of furniture, or impart new skills to your old canine.

Whatever the task, working together on a project with a loved one may strengthen your relationship, produce valuable memories, and give you both something new to anticipate.

•Talk about what intimacy means to you.

When attempting to build intimacy, it is not necessary to wing it.

One easy way to understand how to develop intimacy is to simply talk about it! Share with your lover your ideal time spent together and the activities that strengthen your relationship. Pay heed when they tell you the same thing.

Six
COMMON SEXUAL FANTASIES

Fantasies are fairly common.

Let's start with the fact that everyone has sexual fantasies. Yes, every member of the human species periodically lets their thoughts go to the dark side. Many people feel guilty of their turn ons and erotic fantasies, despite the fact that "no matter what the fantasy is, it's totally fine."

The more we confront sexual fantasy and mainstream the discourse, "we'll beat ourselves up less for having twisted, erotic, hot [thoughts]." That's why we came up with this fantasy crib sheet.

Don't forget to read this section to learn what we're all thinking about in our dirty dreams and how to act them out in reality.

There are seven main categories despite the endless possibilities.

•**Sex with several partners**

Not just you, either. Group sex is the most widely used arousal technique in America.

What makes group sex so alluring? The bulk of people's multi-partner sex fantasies put you in the spotlight. The idea that many people want to have sex with you is a part of the turn on.

Overstimulated states are also brought on by riots, threesomes, and similar events. Imagine this: There are simply more bits, odors, tastes, holes, poles, and sounds in a two-some or solo session.

•**Dominance, control, or immoral sex**

The second most popular fantasy involves bondage, discipline, dominance, and submission (BDSM), as well as sadism and masochism, and it appeals to millions of Americans. Whips and chains are exciting (S&M).

The mutual transfer of power, whether in a sexual or nonsexual situation, is the central premise of BDSM.

The idea of being sexually obedient may be alluring to people who are constantly in power outside of the bedroom. The idea of being in charge may be enticing due to the taboo nature of forced sex and a sense of authority.

This covers the interplay between boss and employee, professor and student, and dad and stepdaughter. Also known as "mock rape," "forced sex" was described in this way.

S&M includes various types of causing or receiving pain, including spanking, whipping, humiliation, and others.

As a result of the play's vulnerability, "truly, this form of play is about radical trust." Such susceptibility also has the capacity to arouse.

•Adventure, novelty, and variety

on a beach or a mountaintop. having fun in a park or using the restroom while wearing a butt plug while boning.

Having sex in a strange location or combining an uncommon sexual action like anal or oral are two examples of how fantasies frequently center on adventure or novelty. Arousal is sometimes associated with the rush of adrenaline that comes with taking a chance and trying something new.

In long-term relationships in particular, it's critical to preserve freshness in order to avoid sexual boredom and maintain an active sex life. Try something new to reignite the passion you shared in the early stages of your relationship.

•Taboos and illegal sex

We yearn for things outside and within the bedroom. It describes how the human brain works. Any sexual activity or behavior that could get us into trouble with the law, or that others might find weird, unlawful, or repulsive in the real world, can be alluring.

Another widespread taboo is worshiping lycra or leather, as well as licking your feet or underarms.

Voyeurism, which involves watching someone have sex without their knowledge or consent, and exhibitionism, which involves exposing one's genitalia in front of others, sometimes with and sometimes without their consent, are the two most common types of forbidden sex.

•Non-monogamy

Open partnerships, polyamory, and swinging are becoming more and more accepted as (healthy and happy!) relationship patterns in addition to being standard masturbation material for those in monogamous relationships.

The majority of people have fantasies about couples who are not monogamous. In other words, one partner has approved of the other's adulterous behavior. Some people have this aspirational non-monogamy.

Others imagine their partners engaging in extramarital affairs. The peculiar dream of discovering your sweetheart having sex with someone else after the fact is known as cuckolding.

•Passion and romance

It seems that romantic cliches such as long beach walks, candlelit dinners, and maintaining eye contact while making love aren't just made up. Every one of these contributes to the fantasy of being desirable, unique, and passionate; "many people want to be treated like kings." Romantic gestures that show a significant expenditure of time, effort, and possibly money might make us feel important to the recipient.

•**Adaptability to erotica**

In this case, two categories stand out:

Gender-bending dreams are more common in those who play with their own gender identity and appearance or who have a spouse who does.

Delusions of sexual fluidity, where the protagonist's sexual orientation appears to be contradicted by the behaviors or characters seen

What makes these so seductive? Playing with different personas and roles may be liberating, creative, and enjoyable. Through it, we can reach a side of ourselves that isn't typically expressed.

Being able to do or be what and who you're not supposed to do or be in your relationship offers a layer of safety and vulnerability that further links us with our spouse. Bending gender roles and orientation also enables people to add something new, novel, and exciting to their sex life while also challenging cultural norms of what you're "supposed" to be or do.

Even while you could glean some insight into what you actually want from others's sexual fantasies, there are a variety of other reasons why individuals have them.

Reasons for fantasizing, from most common to least common

Due to our fascination with different sexual pleasures, our desire to be aroused, our desire to satisfy unmet needs, our desire to escape reality, our desire to explore a sexually taboo desire, our desire to unwind and reduce stress, our desire to feel more sexually confident, and our desire to get ready for a future sexual encounter

How is it that your lover is aware of your fantasies?

It all depends on whether you want to make your fantasy a reality (and it is legal to do so).

Despite the fact that 77 percent of Americans want to communicate their sexual fantasies with a partner, less than 20 percent of Americans have actually done so.

If the behavior is obviously consenting, safe, and legal, and you're prepared to involve your partner(s), the following steps can be helpful:

Detailed prior discussion is required. Then, stay in touch during and after.

- Pick a safe term no matter what kind of imagination you're testing out.
- Continue to engage in safer sex practices.
- Keep going. There's no rush.
- Be open and calm if anything doesn't go according to plan.

A lot of people experience sexual fantasies. You might only be hot for some individuals in your head. You might want to test out some of them in the real world.

If you frequently have sexual fantasies about banned actions and want to explore them in real life, you might want to talk about the cravings with a sex therapist.

If not, take a big breath and talk to your friend. They undoubtedly also have a few sexual fantasies that they'd like to try out in the actual world.

Seven

HOW TO GIVE YOUR PARTNER A HOT SENSUAL MASSAGE

Slow music, gentle touches, and comforting sounds? Sounds and feels fantastic, but imagine giving your partner a sensual massage and feeling their silky skin and sexy parts. Isn't that hot? I just adore giving my husband a sensual massage, and seeing how much he savors it makes me so happy. And I have to admit, I enjoy receiving it as well. Beyond simple relaxation, getting a sensual massage together with your significant other can help you decompress, enjoy sensual pleasure, and strengthen your relationship.

Make sure there is passion in your relationship.

Being able to give a sensual massage is a great way to keep the passion in your relationship alive. I am aware that with time, closeness and passion dwindle as a result of the monotony of many relationships, as well as pressures at work, worries about money, and any other obligations (you name it) divert your focus from the joy of being with that particular someone. However, it is simple to resolve the day's issues and rekindle the desire with a gentle touch. By giving your partner a sensual massage, you not only recreate the fury of your first dates but also make it clear that you value and value your connection with your partner.

The ability to give a sensual massage is a terrific alluring gift for any sweetheart. Whether you massage them just to help them unwind after a hard day or incorporate it in your foreplay, your touch and attention will be more than enough to demonstrate to them that you value and want to be in a relationship with them.

In order to give a passionate, sensual massage, the senses must be awakened.

For the finest benefits, it is essential to awaken the senses before obtaining a sensual massage.

- **Light Lighting is necessary to establish a romantic ambiance.** Draw the curtains, dim the lights, and light some candles to create the perfect atmosphere. The bed needs to be put up and organized because it is the center of the room. Another need is that your mattress shouldn't be too soft. Resistance to the little pressure you'll be applying to specified body regions of your partner is necessary for an effective erotic sensual massage. If the bed is too soft, you'll need to ask the person to move to the floor and use several blankets as cushions.

•Smell

Use the power of aromatherapy to calm the atmosphere so that your seductive, sensual massage can take place. Essential oils offer sexual qualities in addition to relaxing fragrances. Let the aroma permeate the room before your partner enters. Use aroma oils to create scented lotion with calming scents that you may apply to the recipient's body to make your sexually sensuous massage even more unforgettable.

•Sound

You can also include some relaxing music for this special occasion. There is a ton of music available to set this kind of ambiance. Don't discount the fact that music adds dimension to a seductive massage. Still unsure of the perfect song to play to set the right mood?

Don't forget to whisper some foul language into your spouse's ears as you touch them sensually. The atmosphere between you two will be more more private as a result, making the massage even more enjoyable. I understand that it could be frightening to know what to say and how to say it.

•Taste

For each of you to enjoy before, during, or after the exercise, prepare a drink or snack. Throughout your sensual massage, take brief breaks because giving a massage needs a lot of physical effort.

Have some wine or water and some fruits to help you and your partner rehydrate.

•Touch

Make sure your nails are nicely cut and that your skin is warm, not frigid or rough. Your goal of making your lover happy can be accomplished by giving them that extra special touch that can be felt both superficially and deeply in the body.

Tips for swiftly and practically performing a pleasant massage

•A steam bath

It will help you both feel more at ease if you let your mate take a hot bath before the occasion. Allowing the person to undress as they feel comfortable is the next step before settling them on a cozy surface. You might place a towel over the hips just below the tailbone to prevent your full body from being exposed. It produces calming and enjoyable effects.

•Candles scented with massage oil

Slow down when applying oil. Avoid putting it on your partner's body directly. Instead, liberally apply the substance on your hands, rub them together to warm it, and then place your hands on your partner. The massage candle is an excellent tool for lovers who want to engage in intense foreplay as well as for beginners who want to experiment with temperatures in bed. As the massage candle melts, beautiful, warm massage oil is created. Compared to ordinary massage oil, massage candle oil is more comfortable and helps with muscle relaxation because it is already warm, as opposed to having cold oil on your skin. They also have a nice scent, which intensifies the romantic ambiance around you.

•At first, a light touch

Reduce the force of your strokes, especially at first. Even though kneading is great for some types of massage, a sensual massage typically requires considerably softer pressure. Keep your contact light and try to tickle, tease, and stimulate. Circularly swipe your thumb across the back of your spouse.

•Kisses

Remember that you can use your hands and all the other parts of your body as tools in addition to your hands. While kissing your spouse along the spine, gently stroke their hands. One of the finest methods to sustain intimacy in any relationship is by giving each other lots of passionate, regular kisses.

•Look at your partner's physique.

Keep in mind to examine your partner's body as well. Don't restrict your massages to the neck, shoulders, and back, which are hot regions for erogenous zones. Try gently kissing the wrists, blowing on the back of the neck, or nipping the ears. Of course, pay attention to known hot spots for arousal.

•Increasing the heat of the massage

- Massaging the inside of the palm results in a wonderful sensation. Using the pads of your fingertips, draw circles on your partner's hand, moving slowly toward the center, which is the most delicate region. It's worth working up to… Run your fingertips along the edge of the part of the pinkie that is attached to your partner's hand. Ladies, take note: If you want to make it even more passionate, lick and suck his fingers. This will make him swoon over you.

- Gently tap his body with your fingertips from the base of his penis to his navel. With your fingertips, draw a circle around his belly button, widening it as you approach his outside abdomen. In order to avoid tickling him, speed and pressure should be carefully adjusted based on his response because you want to make him groan rather than laugh. Definitely really hot! Doe's it not? The same technique should be used on your girlfriend, males; believe me, our private parts are situated below the belly button, which is a highly sensitive and erogenous place. I'm happy to have you.

- Give your feet a relaxing massage after that. Starting at the ankle, start massaging the oil into the top of the foot. The pad should then be rubbed in a circular motion using your thumbs. Put hard pressure on your companion to stop tickling them.

- As indicated before, when massaging him, utilize your complete body as a weapon rather than just your hands. If you're a woman, stroke his back gently with your breasts before kissing his neck and ears. Men, please pay attention. Slowly lie on top of your lady and stroke her vagina with your penis as you massage her back. Then, give her a sensuous kiss on the back, neck, and other areas of her body.

- At the moment, the skin behind the knees is incredibly fragile and dense with sensitive nerve endings. Your spouse should lie on their stomach and slowly and softly scrape each knee, to slightly warm up the area before sliding your tongue back and forth across the crack.

- Complete the massage by applying pressure adjustments to your partner's inner thighs. The majority of men and women find this area to be sensitive and erogenous, making it difficult to make a mistake with this motion. Add kisses and licks to your massage to make it even more private. When you get to the most delicate spot on the human body, keep caressing, licking, and kissing each other. Now, conjure up some creative ways you two might wish to prolong your sexily private moment:

Making it fun and lighthearted while being willing to try new techniques are the keys to a successful private massage. Find new and creative ways to tickle each other and try to make each other grin, sigh, groan, or scream with delight. The major objective of a massage that is truly enjoyable is to explore one's senses and emotions. Therefore, the most important contribution you can make to this event is your open mind. You're here to explore each other's boundaries and feelings, so be honest with yourself and place as much trust in your partner as you can. A sensual massage is one of the sexiest gifts you can give your partner and it is much more special because it is being provided by someone you deeply care about and love. Your loved one will have a special experience if you do it properly.

Eight

FUN FOREPLAY SEX POSITIONS

When talking about sex positions, we frequently simply address the main action: where to engage in it, how to engage in it, and how to transition from one part of engaging in it to another. The same factors that initially motivated us to engage in foreplay are mostly absent from this discussion. At best, this lapse is reckless; at worst, it is unlawful. After all, without a beginning, there can be no middle and no conclusion. And to be honest, one can't reasonably expect to reach a gratifying conclusion without making at least a little effort in the beginning.

One of the joys of the foreplay position is its innate versatility. Whether you use it to start, end, or insert it in the middle of a statement, it won't ever feel out of place. Although foreplay is not precisely introductory, its objective is that it does not require introduction. Each foreplay position has the potential to be either the opening act or the main event, however many can also serve in either capacity. It is entirely possible to build a broad sexual repertoire with only foreplay positions. However, you'll undoubtedly notice their absence if you try to construct one without utilizing any at all. Of course, some could argue that because there aren't as many foreplay positions, they're more likely to be overlooked. Foreplay can only be performed in a few specific methods, all of which are very self-explanatory. The same could be said about sex in general, though, so yes. Despite the fact that the entire procedure is quite straightforward, we nonetheless develop a few new strategies and go over all of its minute intricacies. If we're willing to put in so much time and effort to get foreplay on, we need to be able to treat it with the respect it deserves. Everything would seem a little flat without it. But when it is, the same set of acts might seem totally brilliant.

•Virgo

The Virgo is the best position for spontaneous oral sex or foreplay that feels a little out of the ordinary. Start out by standing there with your back against a wall. Your spouse should be able to cross their legs and sit across from you if your legs are far enough apart. Next, bend your knees and lean against the wall so your spouse may easily reach your panties. As you start some serious finger and oral play, your partner might even reach around to grip your butt from there.

•Low doggy

The Low Doggy stands on its own because it is so exciting, but it also makes a great lead-in to from-behind penetration. Start by reclining face-down on your bed, a couch, or another comfy surface. As you flex your knees, your feet should be in the air. You are invited to place a pillow under your pelvis to make it a little cozier. So that their head is aligned with your head and their knees are aligned with yours, invite your buddy to climb up onto you. From there, they can jab you with a toy or their fingers. For a little added excitement, they can also grab hold of your hair and pull it.

•**Mirage**

The Mirage is a foreplay position that welcomes participation from both you and your partner. Kneel down with your feet firmly planted on the ground (or a bed, or a couch—you get the picture). Ask your friend to kneel next to you, their backs resting against yours. They can then crouch down to access your genitalia, allowing you full access to theirs in return. Then you can lower yourself onto them and let them start torturing you with their fingers or a sex instrument.

•**Temptation**

The Temptation is a fun method to pump up the heat before, during, or even after sex. A decent place to start is by lying down on the edge of a surface; ideally, it should be fairly high up. Think about a bed (if it's lofted enough), a table, or a countertop. When you're lying down, bend your knees and bring them up to your chest until your feet are quite high in the air. You could even lean a little forward if it's comfortable and support yourself by bending your elbows backward. After that, invite your partner to approach you. While standing, they should be facing you. They can reach down from there and tickle you with their fingers or a toy. They can also stimulate you by reaching up. what is the best? In this foreplay position, you are face to face, allowing for continuous kissing.

•**Reverse**

The Reverse is a fantastic foreplay choice for individuals who want to try something completely new. You should lay down with your knees bent and your feet should be placed in front of you. Just pay attention to what makes you feel safe and at ease. (The bend can be fairly subtle.) Request that your companion lie on top of you. They should be straddling your head while standing with their backs to you and their legs bent. They ought to be looking up. Once there, make the necessary adjustments to bring your partner's genitalia very near your mouth so you may engage in intense oral play.

•**Hunger**

The Hunger is a traditional foreplay position that you'll undoubtedly be familiar with, even if you've never called it that. Start by sitting on the edge of the bed with your knees bent and your toes on the floor. Invite your companion to kneel before you and turn to face you. They can then use their fingers and tongues to play in a variety of ways from there. They can even use a toy to stimulate you if you'd like. Because this position starts on the bed, it's a fantastic entry point into more conventional penetrative sex as well as other types of foreplay.

•Tamer

The Tamer is a highly comforting form of foreplay that is suitable for both drowsy mornings and evenings. To get comfortable, ask your spouse to lie down next to you on their side with their upper body snuggled perpendicular to you between your legs. (You ought to be able to look them in the eyes. If you aren't, one of you is facing the wrong direction! From there, they should have no issue accessing your genitalia, giving them the opportunity to enliven you with their fingers or a sex toy (Dame's Com Wand Vibrator is a great option for this one). And by reaching behind yourself, you can use them.

•Compliment

Anyone can easily add the Compliment, a classic foreplay maneuver, to their sexual toolkit. Ask your partner to kneel just behind the edge of your bed. then descend to your knees before them. Make any necessary changes until you can easily access their genitalia before stimulating them with your mouth, hands, or a sex toy.

•Pendant

The Pendant, often called 69, invites you and your spouse to take equal pleasure in one another. Ask your partner to lie down with their knees bent and their feet in front of them. With your back to them and your legs straddling their chest, you can then climb up on top of them while tucking your head between their knees. From there, you should have limited access to their genitalia and they should have limited access to yours. Ideally, this will give you both the freedom to arouse one another whatever you like—whether that's with your hands, your lips, or a few sex toys.

Nine

HOW TO TALK DIRTY WITH YOUR PARTNER DURING SEX

Dirty talk may initially sound strange as you mull over the best vulgarities to utter to your lover. When it comes to talking dirty, there is uncertainty, thus your comfort level will be more important than your understanding of the topic. Here are some pointers on how to have sexually explicit conversations with your partner as well as tempting things to say to them to up the ante.

•**Go slowly.**

Letting you proceed at your own pace. Nobody except you determines the schedule for acquiring foul language. Texting your dreams may be a preferable option if you're not yet comfortable with any face-to-face action.

•**Pay attention to the things that give you pleasure.**

Being filthy, vulgar, or insulting is not the only definition of dirty speech. "Is it heated to the touch? What it all boils down to is. If a sentence makes you feel sexually excited, it is deemed dirty.

•**Avoid overthinking it.**

You should be able to relate to and flow with your partner's foul language. It doesn't have to be extremely creative; it just needs to feel right to you and your partner. The purpose of "excellent sex" is to be liberated and explorative.

Let nasty talk enhance your sexual experience rather than degrade it. It will be easier to explore the sexual experience the sooner you let go of the pressure you put on yourself.

•**Avoid being overly specific.**

When communicating the problem to your spouse, you do not need to mention their girth or cup size. Something as basic as "I adore your physique" could be the opening line. If you want to use a few, broad words like big, large, and wet work exceptionally well.

•**Relax your partner.**

How comfortable you feel in your relationship is directly impacted by what you're willing to try sexually. "Discussing your interests in filthy language with your partner(s) in advance can be a good strategy to decrease the nervousness while you're actually in the moment," says one expert.

Explore, communicate, and then keep talking. Your relationship will get more intimate as you become more skilled at using dirty language.

•**Stop making snap judgments.**

I constantly tell people to "roll with it and add to it if someone says something a little inappropriate," "have an open mind and have the mindset of 'Yes, and...'," and "be the one who supports someone's sexual fantasy rather than repressing it."

Speaking indecently while having sex.

To spark curiosity:

I'm currently very wet/hard.

I'm not wearing any pants.

I'm getting wet.

I must feel your opposition to me.

I require your lips next to mine.

Wait until we get home, please.

I desire your opinion of myself.

You should fuck me behind if you can.

You should be inside of me.

I want to watch you have fun with yourself.

You should help me undress.

Between my thighs, please.

I wish I could eat you.

Your cock should be in my mouth.

At the very moment:

Grasp me.

Give me a thorough hug.

For me, come.

Kiss my genitalia.

choking me

Seize my ass.

Exactly like that.

That is where.

Tease my hair.

nip me.

Observe me.

Chat with me.

Declare my name.

Speak softly in my ear.

Continue on.

Scream for me.

Kiss my cock.

Make fun of my clit.

Come on over.

You think so?

Identifications:

I love the way you make me feel.

Your cock or puss feels fantastic.

You excel at that.

I adore your physique.

When you clench your teeth and touch me there, I adore it.

When you whisper to me, I adore it.

I adore your moaning.

I adore your sense of taste.

Single-word proverbs:

Slower.

Harder

Louder

Please

More.

Faster.

Deeper.

Fuck.

At the end:

I love how stubborn you can make me.

Your tongue is wonderful.

That was incredible.

Do you want to come back?

Ten

CONCLUSION

I'm delighted you finished reading the earlier chapters; now that you have, I hope you can utilize this book to enhance your sexual and romantic relationships.

I appreciate you reading this book.

YOU ARE UNIQUE.

Printed in Great Britain
by Amazon